for

Margaret & John Michael

with love always

Contents

Foreword

Ten years ago I could make my friend's four-year-old daughter Lily fall asleep by stroking her nose. My friend would praise my skill but I suspect Lily would have fallen asleep had a gorilla stroked her nose. She probably still would, given a dull enough chemistry homework.

So I don't claim any particular skill at massage. Yet I am acutely conscious of the power of touch. You could say I'm envious. As a writer I am painfully aware of the perverseness and artificiality of words when trying to get a message across. Yes they can, with effort, be forced to express complicated, even beautiful things, but for immediacy and potency they're trounced by touch. Touch is the primary human communication.

A friendly hand on a shoulder can convey warmth, security, emotion, the will to heal and a great deal of something this book doesn't mention but that is nevertheless implicit on every page: love. And it does all that quicker than it has taken me to explain it. It does it instantly.

Nobody understands this better than babies. For the first nine months of their existence they know nothing but touch. They've been rolled up in an automatic massage chamber that catered for all their physical needs: the ultimate cuddle.

After all that cosseting the world outside must seem a vast, cold, impersonal place. It would be a crime to stop just because the baby has been born.

All this goes without saying, you may say, but most parents don't massage their babies and a surprisingly large number don't even hold them if they can help it. This doesn't necessarily denote a lack of love; often it is a psychological distancing from the simple enchantment of human contact.

The most common cause is the artificiality of modern life. We think we are super-connected with our mobile phones, emails and "instant" text messages, but we are several stages removed. Nothing connects like touch. What email message can create that common massage condition: bliss?

I know a couple who don't hug their children when they greet them. It's child care by remote control. The mother has told me she doesn't know why she is so inhibited. She would love to learn how to engage with them physically. For parents like her this book is invaluable because it explains as clearly as mere words can, simple procedures for profound contact by way of massage. For the gratuitously tactile it's invaluable too, because it shows the proper way of going about it.

It's all here, from the first touch to the full pumpkin (a massage technique, in case you're wondering).

I wouldn't mind betting that if all babies were massaged there'd be fewer despots in the world. There'd be a lot more Clare Mundys too, which would be no bad thing, for this is a woman who plays Jelly Roll Morton while she works and who can teach an old writer a new word (zugzwang). And she thinks boy babies sometimes need more attention.

As a former boy baby I find that comforting. When I read that Clare had massaged more than 1,000 babies my first thought was "What a lucky woman!" but then I thought "What lucky babies!".

Martin Plimmer
Writer, broadcaster, father of three
and author of the novel exploring
fatherhood: *King of the Castle*

Acknowledgements

I want to thank all the babies with whom I have had the privilege of spending time, and from whom I have learned so much – and their parents for so generously sharing their experiences with me. My thanks also to Melody Weig, my own baby massage teacher at the London College of Massage.

I am truly grateful to Dinedor Books for giving me the opportunity to produce this book; to Rachel Johnson whose design expertise and editorial skills helped bring it to life; to John Wallett for technical and production advice; and to Kim Robson for website design and support.

I would like to thank Tim Neville at the Limelight Family Learning Centre; Pat Russell and Sally Cross of Goldsmith's Community Centre; and Liz, Debbie and Val at Lewisham Pre-School Learning Alliance.

I was helped in my work by Ozzie, who kindly allowed himself to be practised on; by Laura who read the proofs with enthusiasm; by Neil and Steve with research; and, most of all, by Dave whose patience, encouragement and cups of tea have sustained me throughout.

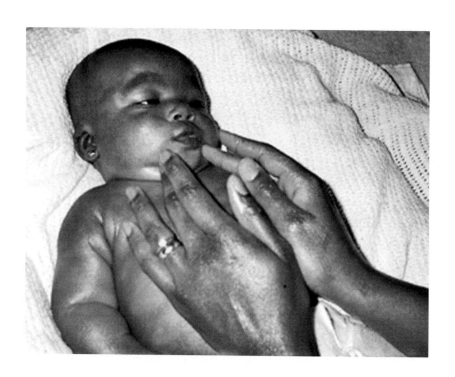

Introduction

Since I became a baby massage teacher in 1992 I have met, massaged and spent the afternoon with more than 1,000 babies. Believe me, they are all different: quirky, funny and unexpected, as individual and unique as you and I.

This book offers practical guidance and advice to help you get the most out of your baby massage sessions, including suggestions on what to try when things do not go according to plan.

If at first you find baby massage hard going, and are tempted to give up, I hope you will be encouraged by the Baby Stories about my encounters with babies who did *not* instantly love being massaged. Like us, some babies simply take longer to let go and relax.

Learning a new skill takes time and patience - and watching your baby learn it with you is just one of the many pleasures of baby massage. In helping parents to discover and enjoy this age-old practice I, too, have learned much about the intriguing ways of babies.

This book is about what I have seen, and what I know.

Note: The information in this book is not intended to replace advice or treatment from your doctor, who should always be consulted if you have any concerns about your baby's health.

For ease of reading, babies are referred to as she or he in alternate sections. All names have been changed to protect the privacy of those too young to give their permission.

a~z of baby massage

adrenalin

Adrenalin is one of the hormones produced in response to alarm and stress: it speeds up the heart rate, dilates the pupils and increases the rate of breathing. Researchers at the University of Wolverhampton have found that a baby's adrenalin levels at birth can be many times higher than those of an adult.

Massage is known to reduce adrenalin and other stress hormones in babies. A gentle version of baby massage can be done right from birth, as it is in India and Malaysia.

See: Recovery from labour

age

How old should your baby be when you introduce baby massage? The answer to this is about personal preference as much as anything: in other words *when you're ready*. A day will come when you feel up to it, or you see a class advertised, or a friend suggests it. Here are my observations about the various ages and stages that babies go through:

premature:

Nurses often massage premature babies while they are in incubators in hospital, because it is now widely accepted that this helps them to gain weight faster, and to recover from the trauma of a difficult delivery. The massage will be gentler than for an older baby, and is generally done for 15 minutes once or twice a day.

newborn

A newborn baby lacks the plumpness for a deep massage, but will certainly benefit from skin contact and stroking, on a daily basis if you want to do it and she enjoys it. The pressure should be just firm enough not to tickle.

1 month

Your baby will benefit from a massage, though if she is still not awake for predictable periods in the day, going to a class may not be possible. You can often find a teacher who will visit you at home.

2 months

She will be awake longer and enjoy seeing new places so now is a good time to go to a baby massage class if you are ready. Your baby will smile and respond to eye contact and attention.

3-4 months

In my experience this is the most usual age range for attending a baby massage class; you have recovered somewhat from the huge upheaval of a new arrival, and your baby is much more alert and interested in her surroundings and in other people.

5 months

Babies of this age are noticeably more sociable: they often respond to other babies with enthusiasm, leaning over to touch and communicate, and will generally interact well with anyone they meet. They are also lovely and plump by now, so there is plenty to grab hold of when you massage.

6-7 months

This is by no means too late to begin baby massage, the only proviso being that if your baby has started to crawl, it may be hard to persuade her to lie down. There are alternative positions you can use if this happens.

See: Older Babies

allergy

When you start using a new product on your baby's skin it is important to keep an eye out for any skin reaction, particularly if your family has a history of allergies (including asthma, eczema or hay fever). This applies to the oil used for baby massage. A ten-minute allergy test carried out on the feet before the first massage is a good precaution.

See: Nut oils

arms

Before birth, the foetal position enables a baby to live in an ever-decreasing space, as well as being an effective protection for the soft vulnerable parts of the body, the stomach, heart, throat and face, which remain hidden. This protective instinct continues for some months after birth, which is why it can be difficult to massage a baby's arms, even by the age of 3 or 4 months.

Some babies will clamp their elbows tightly to their sides when they feel exposed, i.e. lying naked on their back, and you can do nothing to prise those arms free! Not all babies do this, but many will, and it may be impossible to do more than just stroke the outsides of your baby's arms until she feels ready to relax and let go.

It will encourage this process if you only attempt to uncurl one arm at a time, leaving the other one clamped. Coaxing it gently away from the side of her body with soothing strokes and sounds may persuade your baby that there is nothing to fear. Often a baby will only ever 'release' one arm during a massage, keeping the other for her own use, to wave about, grab hold with, or suck on.

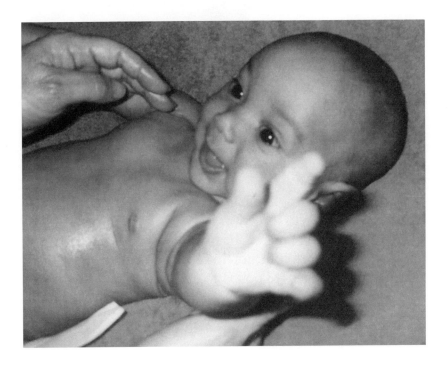

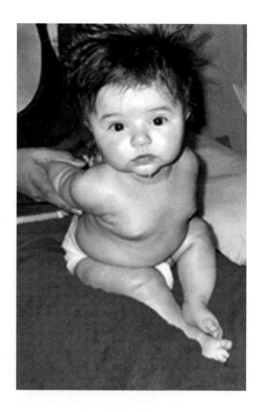

asthma

While there is a genetic factor involved in susceptibility to asthma, exposure to infection in early life also seems to be influential. For instance it has been known for some time that asthma is more common in first-born children, possibly because they are less exposed to germs from siblings.

Research has found that older children who are massaged show an improvement in their asthma.

awake

When you choose your time for baby massage, make sure your baby is wide-awake. This goes for you, too. It is not generally a good idea to massage your baby at bedtime because massage is stimulating and may wake your baby up rather than send her to sleep.

It is not good practice to massage your baby while she is sleeping, but it may occasionally happen if you attend a massage class that your baby has decided to sleep through, and you want to have a go at one or two strokes. However, being massaged while you sleep is an invasion of your privacy! Don't be surprised if your baby is cross, should she waken up.

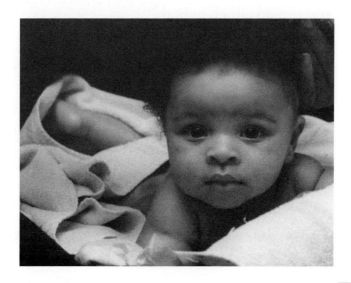

back massage

If you massage your baby while he is naked, his back will be the biggest surface area of his body, so this is a good stroke to use at the end of the massage. With your baby lying across your lap, or lengthways, stroke from the back of his head all the way down, including his buttocks and legs, right down to his feet. This should be a slow, smooth sweep, repeated over and over. The repetitive rhythm of this movement can have a soporific effect on you both, like stroking a cat.

Stroking *down*wards from the head is soothing and calming.

Stroking *up*wards from the feet or the lower back is stimulating and enlivening.

You can do either, or both.

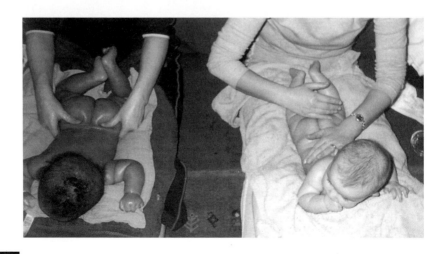

banana

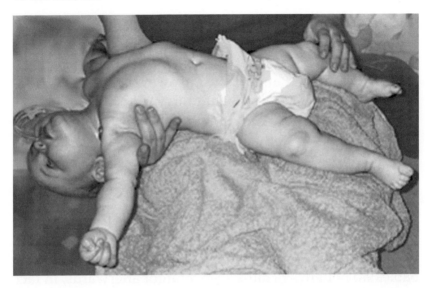

This is my name for a simple back-bend, part of the more active flexing and stretching movements that can be added to your baby massage routine. To do the Banana stretch, place your baby's lumbar curve (the middle part of his back) across your legs while you are sitting on the floor, and then gently encourage a backwards stretch. In this position your baby's head and legs counterbalance each other.

Some babies love this position and will voluntarily drop their head backwards and gaze at the room upside-down. It gives a lovely stretch to all the muscles down the front of the body.

See: Pumpkin

bath time

Whilst it is a good idea to get into a daily bath-and-bedtime routine, this is not necessarily the best time to give a massage. It is tempting to connect the two, since at bath-time your baby will be naked and playful. However, there are a few reasons why I don't recommend this.

Firstly, by the evening your baby is starting to get tired so you need to encourage a winding-down process rather than the stimulating effects of a massage. Secondly, you too are probably tired, which is not ideal when giving a massage.

Thirdly, you don't want to get tied up in a situation where your baby will *only* fall asleep with a massage, because this will not always be convenient or possible. And fourthly, babies do not always fall asleep straight afterwards, in fact quite the contrary sometimes, since massage has a stimulating effect initially.

See: Playtime

birth trauma

Unfortunately the experience of being born is not always straightforward and simple. Whether during labour itself, or in the immediate aftermath, there can sometimes be distress for the baby and a recovery period will follow during which you and your baby will need time to recuperate.

During this period your baby may sleep a great deal, or may be very jumpy and startled by everything around him. He may react to any change from one state to another, (e.g. being dressed or undressed) by crying, and require a lot of soothing and holding to calm him down.

Massage can be a good way to encourage your baby to relax and let go of the tension that he may still have in his body as a result of stressful experiences. Touching and stroking have an effect on hormone levels, boosting those that make us feel good and reducing stress hormones such as adrenalin.

See: Baby story - birth trauma
        Health benefits
        Recovery from labour

birth trauma

George was born slightly premature, with the cord wrapped around his neck. His distress had been prolonged, and he had had to be given emergency resuscitation and placed in the special care baby unit after delivery.

His mother and grandmother were present when I arrived. His mother Jill said they didn't know if baby massage could help George, but they wanted to "find something to calm him down". Jill told me George, who was now 2 months old, had been rushed to hospital three times with breathing problems since he was born, and each time there had been no medical reason for the problem.

George was a small baby, wrapped up in a shawl and with his eyes tightly shut. Right away I noticed that his breathing was rapid and huffy, as though he was panting. I sat with Jill and her mother Marie and we talked for a while about Jill's experiences of labour and delivery. I explained that I would show them the baby massage routine on George and then Jill could take over from me. We unwrapped and undressed George, but placed a folded towel across his stomach with just his legs and arms uncovered, and I started to massage his feet.

baby story

After a few moments George opened his eyes. The massage proceeded as far as his chest, but no further: at this point his breathing became faster and it seemed like he was having a panic attack. Panic breathing causes an imbalance of oxygen and carbon dioxide because the mouth is open and too much air is taken in; one remedy is to breathe into a paper bag, but clearly this would not be appropriate for a baby.

I wrapped him up again in his shawl, and then placed both my hands on his arms and rocked him very gently, speaking to him in a soft voice. If he had a memory of the neck constriction he had experienced at birth, and was afraid of it happening again, aversion to being touched anywhere near that area would be a natural instinct.

I suggested to Jill that she keep him covered with a towel, and massage only his feet and hands to start with, gradually including his legs and arms, but proceeding very slowly. Gradually she could move on to his chest, head and back, but only once he was accustomed to the feeling of being massaged. continued...

baby story continued...

I saw George again two months later, and he was a different baby. Jill told me that at first she had spent a lot of time just holding his feet and talking to him. There had been no more panic breathing episodes, and he was now much more active when she massaged him, kicking his legs and holding on to her fingers sometimes, "as if he's telling me not to stop".

When a baby's first experiences of being touched are traumatic and frightening it can take a lot of patience to persuade him to accept stroking and massage touch without fear. To begin with, just holding and talking is enough.

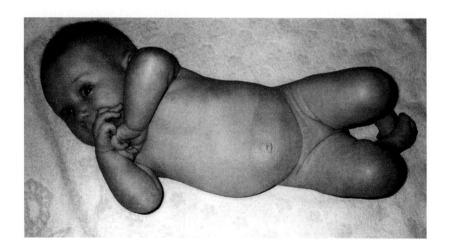

bliss

One of the best after-effects of baby massage is the state called 'quietly alert' when a baby will lie contentedly awake, in a sort of trance, not needing or wanting anything more. This seems very similar to the calm state of mind and body following meditation or hypnosis, in which heart rate and pulse are lowered and the whole system is at peace. In Buddhism this is the condition called bliss.

Research has shown that regularly massaged babies spend longer periods being quietly alert.

boys

Contrary to general assumption, boy babies are more vulnerable from birth than girls, and lag behind them developmentally by 4 to 6 weeks. Research indicates that boy babies sometimes get less physical contact and cuddles than they need: maybe unconsciously we encourage and value their independence more.

Massage is a great way to give boy babies the physical attention they need for social confidence and brain development.

chestiness

Chestiness, snuffles and a blocked nose result from congestion caused by an excess of mucus, Nature's ingenious way of ridding the body of germs. If you are worried that your baby's blocked nose will prevent her 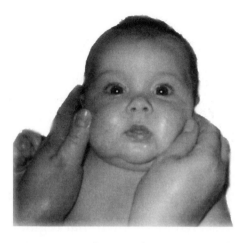 from breathing when she's asleep, lay her on her side, with a rolled-up towel to prevent her rolling backwards, and one nostril will soon clear.

Another way to clear a blocked nose is to stroke down each side of your baby's nose with your thumbs. Stroking across and above her eyebrows and over her cheekbones just below the eye sockets will work on the sinus areas. All these strokes should be slow, but firm.

Percussion (firm tapping using a cupped hand) across the upper back will relieve chestiness, and can be used on older children as well as babies. Ideally her chest, shoulders and head should be sloping downwards, while you tap.

circulation

Babies do not have good circulation so their hands and feet may feel chilly even on a warm day or in a warm room. Massage is an effective way to bring blood to the extremities, starting with your baby's feet, which should be thoroughly warmed up before you move on to her legs.

If your baby is inexplicably grumpy during the massage, check that the room is warm enough and she is not lying in a draught.

See: Room temperature

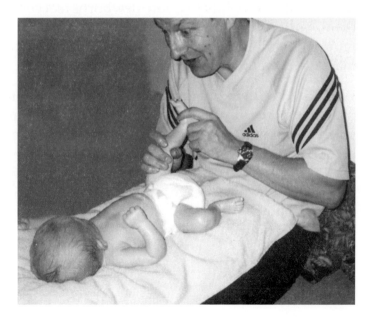

colic

Ruth and Simon were at their wits' end with their baby Lily, who was two months' old and screaming when I arrived. While Ruth and I talked, Simon paced around the downstairs rooms with Lily, still screaming. "It's always like this," Ruth told me. "Either she's asleep, briefly, or feeding, or screaming. We've tried the usual colic remedies but nothing helps."

I admired the lambswool fleece Ruth's mother had sent over from Australia for Lily to lie on; newborns feel cosy lying on them, but unfortunately it wasn't helping the colic. Simon returned with Lily, and I suggested trying to do some baby massage even though she was still screaming.

We laid Lily down on a pillow but kept her covered apart from her stomach, and I placed my hand on her abdomen, which felt almost rigid. I circled my hand slowly clockwise across her whole stomach, repeating the circle over and over while Lily continued to scream. It was an unnerving experience! Ideally massage is a mellow and relaxing process, but for a baby with severe colic it is a therapy applied at a time of desperate need.

baby story

I massaged Lily for only fifteen minutes, after which we wrapped her up once more and Simon took her out of the room, still screaming. But he came back shortly after, looking a bit dazed, and said she had fallen asleep in his arms and he had put her down in her cot. This was clearly an unusual experience for all three of them.

I followed up the visit with a phone call the next day, and Ruth told me Lily had slept for five hours that night, which was apparently a record so far, and they were very much convinced that baby massage was the reason. Because it works deep on the central nervous system, a powerful effect takes place that may not be obvious straight away. Lily had not noticeably relaxed during her massage, but had clearly been affected some time afterwards.

colic

Colic is unmistakable. Wind can be painful and cause crying, but colic pain is severe and causes screaming. This commonly happens in the evening and can be prolonged.

The bad news about colic is that no-one really knows what it is, why some babies get it, or how to prevent it. There are some remedies you can try, such as warm baths for your baby, and holding her in a more upright position when you feed her.

While breastfeeding avoid sorbitol, found in apple juice, as this is now known to upset babies' digestion. Drink grape juice instead; also fennel or chamomile tea may help.

The good news is that babies grow out of colic, usually by around 12 weeks. The other good news is that massage can really help. The strokes to use are:

> Stomach massage
>
> Back massage
>
> Waterwheel

All these can be done through clothing, and must be reasonably firm to have an effect.

See: Colic - baby story
      Cranial osteopathy

constipation

This can be a problem when you start to introduce solids. A gentle massage of the stomach slowly in a clockwise direction is effective. Also useful is to hold your baby's bent knees and push them towards her stomach: two or three pushes in rapid succession, pause, then repeat.

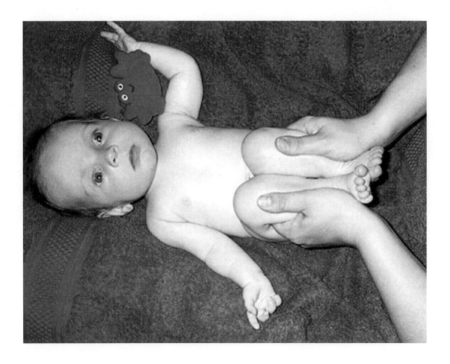

contra-indications

There are a few situations when a baby either should not be massaged, or special care should be taken:

- Raised temperature

- After recent surgery

- On broken or infected skin

- On an immunization site, or following an injection if the baby is unwell

- When the baby is taking medicine

- Unstable joints, brittle bones or fracture

- If the baby is tired or lethargic

There is a view that babies should not be massaged before their six or eight week health assessment, because there may be doubt about the stability of the hip joints.

Since babies in other cultures are massaged right from birth, this may be unnecessarily cautious. The flex and stretch exercises involving the legs may be omitted until after this check.

Babies with congenital dislocation of the hip can, however, be massaged according to Amelia Auckett, a nurse and baby massage teacher, who recommends it as an important sensory stimulation that helps such babies to catch up when they become mobile again.

cranial osteopathy

Also known as Paediatric Osteopathy, this therapy seems to have very beneficial results for babies suffering from a variety of common ailments, including the after-effects of a difficult birth. It is based on the idea that the skull is not rigid but continually expands and contracts in a pulsing motion, which helps the flow of cerebro-spinal fluid. This fluid protects and nourishes the brain and spinal cord, and removes waste products.

The birth process can trap cranial nerves and leave a baby with discomfort, similar to a persistent headache. Babies and children are treated for such ailments as asthma, eczema, colic, behavioural problems and sleep disorders.

I have heard directly from mothers that cranial osteopathy has helped the following:

- The baby's head always turning to one side because of the position the baby was in during delivery

- The baby not liking her head to be touched or stroked, crying or pulling away

- Generalised and frequent crying for no apparent reason, this becoming obvious only after she and her mother spent time in a group with other babies

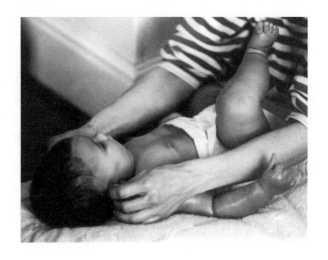

- After a difficult delivery, including caesarian

- Sleep disturbances

- Feeding problems

See: Baby story - feeding

crying

While many babies take to massage easily and straight-forwardly, for others massage is an intense experience that needs to be introduced gradually in small amounts. If your baby cries at first, lots of patience is recommended.

Alison brought Patrick, her third child, to his first baby massage class when he was 10 weeks old. He started to cry as soon as she undressed him, and didn't stop until she wrapped him up in the towel and walked about the room soothing him. She spent most of the class observing the others.

At the second class Patrick accepted just a few minutes of massage before starting to cry loudly and vigorously. Throughout the third class he cried intermittently, with several short interludes of massage. Alison said she was trying to massage him at home too, and that he was starting to like having his feet and legs massaged.

By the fourth class Patrick was calmer and accepted most of the massage but still had a prolonged crying episode towards the end of the session. But at our fifth and final class we were amazed at the transformation: Patrick lay very contentedly on his back and then happily on his front,

baby story

smiling and looking around at the other babies while Alison massaged him. For the first time he did not cry once.

It was so interesting to see Patrick gradually lose his fear and resistance over the weeks. It would have been so easy to give up, but Alison was convinced of the benefits of massage because she could see other babies in the class enjoying it, and she persisted.

It is a mystery why some babies cry like this. Sometimes a baby needs coaxing, reassuring and encouraging: it took Patrick five weeks to get used to the new sensations of massage, with lots of short feeds and cuddles in between, but he got there eventually

crying

Entire books are available on the subject of crying babies! I am only concerned here with what to do if your baby cries *during massage*. There are two types of crying that may occur at some point, neither of which indicates that your baby hates being massaged, or hates *you*.

1. Real crying:

   Your baby is telling you she needs something so stop the massage and feed, change, let her take a nap or whatever. You may be able to continue the massage later.

2. Pretend crying:

   Your baby is bored, grumpy or wants attention; you can usually sort it out just by doing something different, like sitting her up for a look around, rocking her or giving her a cuddle. Continue the massage once she has cheered up again.

depression: post-natal

Post-natal depression can affect anyone, and medical help should be sought because there are helpful treatments available. Complementary therapies may be able to help the hormonal imbalance thought to be the cause.

Research carried out by paediatrician Dr Yvette Glover found that doing baby massage helps mothers to recover faster from post-natal depression, and has a very positive effect on the relationship between a mother and her baby. Learning and practising baby massage is a good way to relax and enjoy your baby, and attending a class gives social contact and support.

difficult baby

See: Sensitive baby

digestion

Massage can assist in a baby's digestive processes and ease related problems such as wind and constipation. Massage his stomach always in a clockwise direction, as this follows the path of the large intestine and will encourage wind to be eliminated.

If your baby is regurgitating his milk, try feeding him in a more upright position rather than lying down, as gravity will ensure the food enters the lower part of his stomach straight away. This will also satisfy your baby's hunger more rapidly.

disability

There is a special place for massage in the life of a baby who is born with, or develops, a physical or other disability. Such babies enjoy and benefit from the reassurance of touch through massage, and it is an ideal way for a parent, by relaxing, to let go of some of the intense anxiety they are likely to be experiencing.

For children with impaired verbal skills, touch is a powerful alternative means of communication – massage can help in the release of frustration, anger or sadness for a child who cannot express these emotions in words.

Autistic spectrum children may respond well to giving, as well as receiving, massage. For older children this can be done through clothing, and kept to short ten-minute sessions. Massage on the back, hands and feet is enough.

I worked with Frances and her baby Ruby, who was suspected of having hearing loss. During her massages Ruby maintained good eye contact and Frances told me that giving Ruby a daily massage helped her to feel, literally, *in touch* with her baby.

draughts

How delightful it must be to emerge from the perfectly regulated temperature of the womb into a hot climate, one in which a light warm breeze wafting across your skin merely adds to the comfort.

Understand that the opposite is also true: in a warm room, even the teeniest cold draught can ruin a baby's experience of massage. Before you begin the massage remove your shoes and socks, and wear a sleeveless or short-sleeve top: this will help you detect the draughts that can seep in under doors and round your window frames.

dry skin

Babies often have patches of dry skin where they have dribbled, or where milk has dripped and then dried. Commonly these are just behind the ear lobes and in the creases of the neck. During a baby massage session, dab some oil into these areas with one finger, and then rub it in until it is absorbed. Massage is the ideal way to apply creams or ointments that you may have been prescribed for your baby's dry skin.

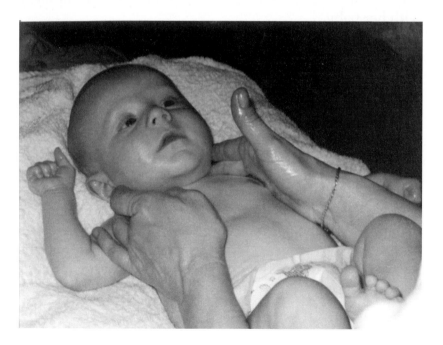

eczema

As well as massaging many babies with eczema, I suffered from it badly myself as a young child. The good news is that babies with eczema often grow out of it eventually, and will have no memory of the sore skin, itching and broken sleep.

During a massage I have found it helpful to cover the baby's tummy with a cotton or muslin square to discourage her from scratching while I massage her legs and arms, and then to hold her arms gently out of the way while massaging her tummy. Even a towel can cause itching, so spread a smooth fabric such as a cotton sheet on top of it.

You may have been prescribed special cream or ointment to use on your baby's skin and in her bath, called oilatum. You can use this instead of oil for baby massage. Dry skin conditions benefit from frequent moisturizing, so you can massage your baby twice a day if she is willing.

Eczema is a condition that is aggravated by heat. When you massage your baby it helps to keep the room coolish, though not draughty.

equipment

There are some essential items you will need to massage your baby, and some optional extras you might like to include:

oil

The types of oil are described under section O. It is easier to use oil from a shallow dish than straight from the bottle because your hands will be slippery once you get started. Any oil left over should be disposed of, not used again.

towel

Oil is messy! A large (bath size) towel will protect your clothing as well as the surface you are massaging on. I don't recommend lying your baby directly on waterproof material such as a changing mat because it is slippery and non-absorbent, and also because it is not warm and comfortable to lie on.

support

You will need a pillow to lie your baby down on, and you may like to use a small cushion to raise her head a little so she can see you. To protect your back from strain, and relax your upper body, you also need support to lean against while you are massaging her.

These extras will add to the atmosphere and help your baby to associate massage with many pleasurable sensations:

light

Babies will gaze fixedly at any bright light source, so subdued lighting will make it easier to get eye contact with your baby, and help you both to relax and concentrate.

music

There are two good reasons for playing a tape or CD while you massage: if you are alone with your baby it breaks up the silence, and if you are massaging with a group of friends with babies it can help drown out some of the noise.

aroma

As well as touch and sound, don't forget scent: massage is about stimulating all the senses. Essential oils are not recommended for massaging babies younger than six months, so instead you might like to add two drops to your towel or use a vaporizer in the room.

exercise

Exercise and yoga classes are developing for mothers with their babies, in which babies are introduced to a range of physical movements. There is a view that babies in the West do not get enough exercise, spending too much time strapped into car seats and prams or lying down.

This opinion is based on the experience of women in the Western Amazon, who climb and move about with their babies, and on the idea that many babies get too much sensory and too little physical stimulation: well-exercised babies sleep better and more regularly, and cry less.

If your baby is very active and energetic, or for older babies who don't want to lie down for long, a baby massage session can include some fun exercises that can be added during or at the end of the massage. Two examples in this book are the forward and backward bends described in Banana and Pumpkin

See: Yoga

eye contact

Baby massage is not at all like an adult massage, during which you lie still and usually have your eyes closed. Babies will *not* lie still, and they love to interact with you, chiefly through eye contact and facial expression.

Babies who were shown a video picture of their mother with her eyes closed became upset, indicating that eye contact is very important to babies, who can become disturbed if it is deliberately withheld. Even newborn babies can focus on an object or face – the best distance is 12 inches away from their eyes.

From the start of the massage maintain eye contact with your baby as you proceed; if there is another person present keep your attention on your baby, because she will certainly notice if you get distracted. Not only will she become upset if you look away for long, but she will feel the change in the quality of your touch if your attention lapses.

All massage is an intimate process of communication without words, involving trust and presence. Eye contact will show your baby that you are truly involved.

See: Baby story – eye contact

eye contact

Eye contact is one of the most powerful signalling devices we possess, indicating interest, attention, love and sometimes hostility or intimidation. Because babies cannot understand language, eye contact is one way we can reassure and communicate with them while massaging. Imagine how you might feel if someone you were having a conversation with consistently refused to look at you. The primary reaction is to think *something's wrong,* and often *something's wrong with me.*

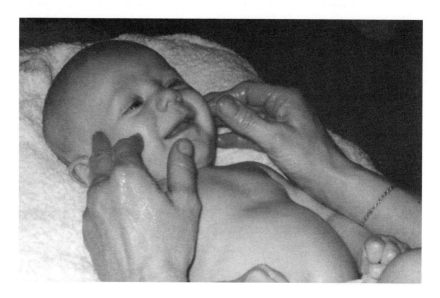

baby story

From very early on, babies engage in eye contact quite naturally. I had a very disturbing experience when I visited a baby whose parents were in the throes of packing up their house for a move. We took the baby into the bedroom so I could teach massage, and her mother and I sat on the bed. As I always do at the start of a session, I held the baby up so we could look at each other, and spoke to her in a soft voice, introducing myself and telling her what we were going to do.

But this baby would not meet my eyes. She kept her head still while her eyes darted from side to side as though she was watching a tennis match, and no matter where I moved her I could not get her to look at me. After a while I offered to pass the baby to her mother so that I could observe their interaction, but the mother resisted. I never did find out why this baby wouldn't make eye contact, but it was the only time I've ever met a baby who wouldn't.

face

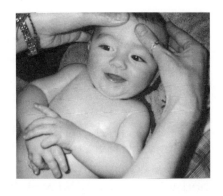

Some babies are not keen on having their face massaged, so you may have to proceed cautiously and do a little bit to start with. It is not essential to massage the face, though it is nice to include it if possible. Wipe your fingers on the towel first, as oil is not necessary, and be especially careful not to get oil near his eyes.

Stroke firmly across the brow and eyebrows, down both sides of the nose and across the cheekbones. Stroke above and below the lips and under the chin, and then circle the cheeks.

Some babies love to have their ears massaged: stroke all around the outside edge, including soft pinching movements, and stroke a little bit of oil behind the ear lobes where the skin can get dry. Finally dip your fingers in oil and stroke them from the back of the neck round to the front, getting into the creases.

feeding

If your baby gets hungry during his massage, stop and wrap him in the towel while you feed him. Afterwards resume the massage unless your baby has fallen asleep.

When I teach a class plenty of time is allowed for the interruptions of feeding and naps, but at home you can choose a time when this is less likely to happen.

I have encountered a few babies in my classes who had feeding problems, i.e. were unwilling to feed for more than a few moments at a time. A simple remedy was found for this problem.

See: Baby story – feeding

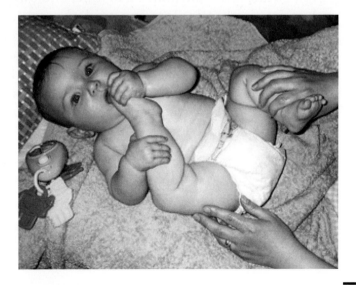

feeding

Two babies attended my classes who were experiencing feeding problems. Jasmine's baby Sally had a happy temperament and was alert and responsive, but she was not gaining weight as she should, and some weeks she was losing weight. Jasmine said the doctors she had seen didn't take her seriously when she told them Sally refused to feed, and that she had given up breastfeeding, reluctantly, in the hope that bottle-feeding would help her baby to gain weight.

I watched Jasmine as she attempted to feed Sally. The baby would swallow a small amount of milk, and then turn away and resist the bottle. Jasmine said she could see what enjoyment other babies and their mothers had from feeding, and she was sad to be missing out on that. She said she had been advised to force feed Sally by holding her head firmly in place while the bottle was in her mouth, but as I watched her try this, Sally just coughed and spluttered, and it was a miserable experience for them both.

I thought Sally might be helped by cranial osteopathy, and Jasmine was willing to try alternatives. A couple of weeks later they returned to the baby massage class, and Jasmine reported that Sally was now taking proper feeds and starting to regain weight. The cranial osteopath had discovered

baby story

that the powerful force of the ventouse delivery had not just pulled on Sally's head, but also on her diaphragm, which had lifted out of position and was preventing the flow of milk reaching her stomach. The two treatments he gave her effectively put this back in place, and from then on Sally was able to keep her feed down.

~

Julia's baby Zac had a similar problem following a ventouse birth: his cardiac valve, through which food passes from the oesophagus to the stomach, had become distorted and Zac was not able to keep his milk down. In adults a cardiac valve that is not closing properly results in indigestion and painful acid reflux, as stomach acid leaks into the gullet. Julia had been told to keep Zac mostly in an upright position, and was massaging him propped up on two pillows.

Cranial osteopathy helped to return Zac's cardiac valve to a one-way system, allowing milk to pass through to his stomach without being regurgitated.

feet

The first time you massage your baby with oil it is a good idea to work on his feet for about ten minutes at the start, to see whether there is a skin reaction. This is extremely rare, and the remedy is very simple. If you notice excessive redness, especially if your baby's feet remain cool, all you need to do is wash off the oil using soap and water, and try a different oil.

If you always begin the massage with your baby's feet, he will soon be able to recognise what you are doing as the routine becomes familiar to him.

You may have noticed that your baby's hands and feet are often cooler than the rest of his body, even in warm conditions. This is because babies do not have good circulation, so massage is an excellent way to get blood flowing to the extremities. Work on your baby's feet until they are warm before you move on to his legs. Just holding and enclosing his feet will begin the warming process.

frequency

In research terms, a 'regularly massaged' baby means one who has been massaged two or three times a week over a period of months. Premature babies however may receive two or three short (5 or 10 minute) massages every day whilst they are in hospital.

In countries where baby massage is traditional, the baby is massaged every day. Not only that, but when a baby is delivered by a midwife she will massage both baby *and* mother daily for the first ten days or so. This seems a very enlightened way to minimize the exhaustion and stress of those early days, and possibly also reduce the incidence of post-natal depression.

I suggest a daily massage when you first learn the techniques, because practice will help both you and your baby to familiarize yourselves with the strokes; you will also find out his particular favourites, and what, if anything, he doesn't care for.

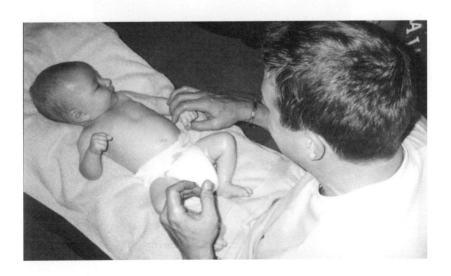

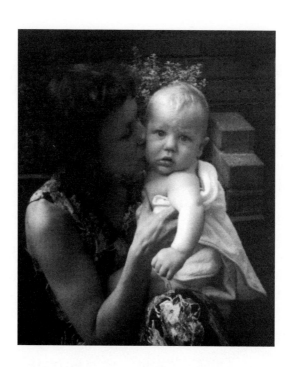

grapeseed oil

This is one of the recommended oils for baby massage, and the one I use most often in my classes. Grapeseed oil does not have a strong scent, is edible, and is easily absorbed by the skin. It is lighter and less viscous than olive oil, and is generally available in supermarkets.

See: Oils

growth

One of the most widely accepted research findings on baby massage showed that premature babies who were massaged three times a day for ten days gained nearly 50% more weight and were discharged from hospital six days earlier than the norm.

Massage is known to influence activity in the vagus nerve (part of the autonomic nervous system) which stimulates food absorption. Incidentally, this nerve is also responsible for hiccups, which babies often seem to get during a massage.

gut

The gut (meaning stomach and intestines) is a large and complex part of the human system. It has been found that neurotransmitters in the brain connect our emotions to the stomach, perhaps explaining the common terms that link our feelings to this part of the body, such as *gut reaction, fed up* etc.

Babies have complex responses to being massaged in this area, perhaps because it has a powerful link to the way they feel, not just physically but emotionally too.

Even though your baby may cry the first time you massage her stomach, it is an important area with a lot of activity going on and it is worth persisting on another occasion.

See: Stomach

hands

The massage routine includes your baby's hands, and at times when it is not convenient to undress your baby for a full body massage there will be many occasions when you can stroke and massage just his hands and fingers.

If you have ever had your hands massaged you will know how soothing and relaxing this can be. Because our hands and fingers contain so many nerve endings they have the sensitivity to identify and distinguish between many shapes and textures, and are very responsive to being stroked.

The instinct to keep the fingers tightly curled is a good protection for delicate little fingers; they may be coaxed to uncurl if you stroke the inner wrists.

It may seem obvious, but make sure your own hands are thoroughly warmed up before you start baby massage!

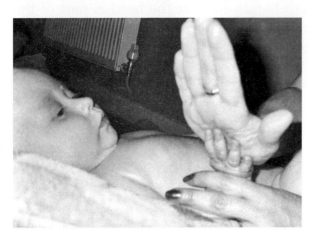

head

Now that babies are put on their backs to sleep as protection against cot death, there is an increased incidence of squashed or flattened heads, usually caused by the head flopping to one side during sleep. A neck support to keep your baby's head from slipping sideways when he is asleep may help.

I have been told by African and Caribbean women that one of the reasons for doing baby massage is "to make the head a nice shape" after birth. Ventouse delivery can also result in a misshapen head.

If your baby consistently cries whenever you touch his head, he might be experiencing some discomfort in the head or neck. The compression caused by labour can sometimes affect the nerves in this region, which is easily corrected by the gentle movements of cranial osteopathy.

Stroking with both hands all over the head is part of the massage routine, and I also include tapping with the soft pads of your fingers, either together or in a wave-like motion. Try this on your own head to discover the strangely soothing "raindrop" sound it makes.

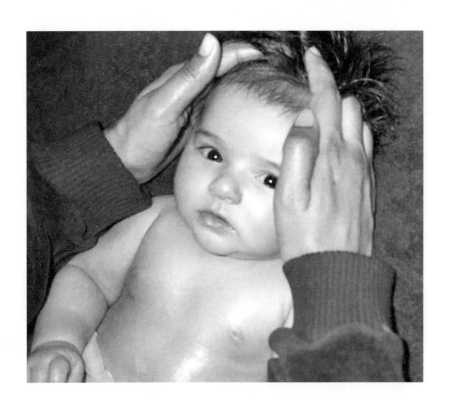

health benefits

Research in Britain and the USA has shown the following benefits for babies who are massaged regularly (at least 3 times a week) and their mothers.

- Better food absorption and weight gain

- Longer times of being 'quietly alert'

- Fall asleep in less than 10 minutes, while the average is 22 minutes

- Reduced colic and teething pain

- Improved stress response to inoculations

- In baby *and in mother*, massage increases oxytocin (a hormone that promotes emotional attachment) and reduces cortisol (a stress hormone)

- Baby massage results in lowered blood pressure and less need for medication *for the person giving the massage*.

See: Appendix - research sources

hug

After you have massaged your baby's arms, if he has let go and they are relaxed and floppy you can cross them over his chest so that he gives himself a hug. Some babies find this rather amusing, in which case you have a little game to be played over and over.

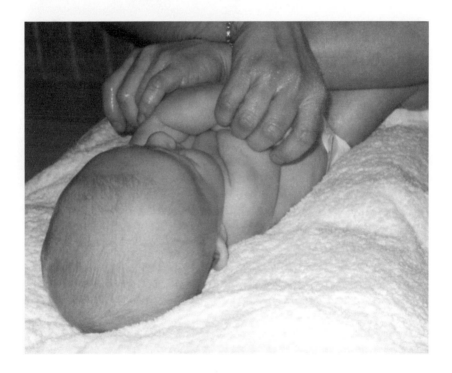

humour

Is there anything quite so mysterious and irresistible as a baby's sense of humour? Or anything as delightfully surprising as discovering what it is that makes your own baby burst into a merry fit of chuckles at the tender age of 12 weeks? Babies seem to develop a sense of the absurd very early on, long before they can walk, talk, crawl, or sit up.

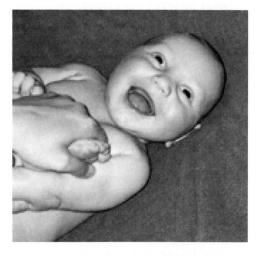

There may be debate about when babies first 'really' smile, but laughter is beyond doubting. In the massage class a baby will sometimes laugh outright at one of the more active movements, such as the hug, or when massaged around their shoulders and neck. Absurdly, I get the impression the baby is surprised, which implies they expected things to go *this* way when suddenly they went *that* way.

Expectations at 12 weeks old? Absurd!

inoculations

Research shows that massaged babies react with less stress to injections. This does not necessarily make it less stressful for you!

Fears and phobias are easily passed on to children. If you know you are likely to be upset when your baby gets her jabs, either look away, or ask a nurse to hold her for you while you wait outside the room. This will not traumatize your baby; most babies are fretful and grumpy for the rest of the day in reaction to inoculations.

interruptions

Interruptions should be kept to an absolute minimum by turning off your phone and choosing a time when you can dedicate half an hour or more to your baby in peace and quiet. When doing massage, it is a good principle to keep one hand always in contact with your baby's skin, for example while you scoop up some more oil. Removing both hands at the same time can be disorienting.

intimacy

Touching another person's body is one of the most intimate forms of human contact, and should only be done with respect and permission. You may think this doesn't apply to babies – after all, they are helpless and depend on you for every bodily need – but when it comes to massage it is still important to respect your baby's feelings.

Sometimes she will not be in the right mood for a massage, and will make this known in no uncertain terms. I'm not talking about a short period of settling down, and maybe some grizzling; babies often complain when you take off their clothes, and then complain again when you put them back on, because babies don't generally like the transitions between one activity, or state of being, and another.

Before you commence massage it's good practice to ask permission, verbally and with eye contact, even though you may not be sure if you get a definite 'yes' or 'no'. This acknowledges the profound intimacy of massage and reminds you that it is something you do *with*, and not *to*, your baby.

Touching someone's skin, being close, looking into each other's eyes and exchanging words and sounds - all these are an essential part of love and communication, and you are teaching your baby some very important things about security and being cared for, as well as sharing with her the pleasure of movement and relaxation.

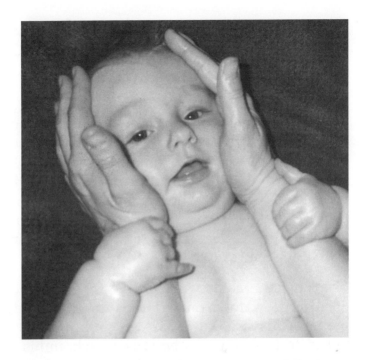

Conversely, there is something very uncomfortable about being touched by someone who is looking elsewhere, thinking about other things, or chatting to another person without paying much attention to *you*. So, when you massage your baby, make sure she knows that during this special time with you she is the centre of the universe.

See: Baby story - intimacy

intimacy

Matthew was eight months old when I first went to teach baby massage to his parents, who were both present. This is quite a bit older than usual for starting massage, so I wasn't sure if he would be willing to lie or sit still. Matthew was a very alert, lively baby who was already crawling. His father Don and mother Janine were reading to him every day and told me he was very aware and seemed to understand everything they said to him.

I explained to Matthew what we were going to do, and he obediently lay down on his back and very happily allowed me to demonstrate the massage strokes to his parents. I talked to Matthew and he talked back, in his own baby language, very readily; it was obvious that he was used to conversations, and highly articulate.

But when Janine took over the massage, within ten minutes Matthew was complaining and making a fuss, and I had to laugh as Janine and Don turned to me looking puzzled. There they both were, one on either side of their beloved son, eager to do their best for him and clearly succeeding, until this moment. However, instead of focusing their attention quietly on Matthew, they had lapsed into an animated conversation between themselves. Poor Matthew evidently felt ignored and was having none of it.

baby story

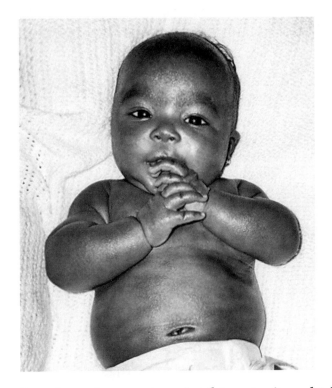

It took an observer to point this out, after which the massage went well. Babies are more sensitive to our behaviour than we realize; although they cannot always have our undivided attention, they are entitled to it during baby massage.

jaw

Your baby's jaw is very busy the whole time he is awake, sucking, crying, gnawing on his fist or any other objects within reach, and making all sorts of 'talking' noises. He will copy the way your mouth looks if you say words slowly in front of him.

All these activities can result in a build-up of tension in the jaw, which will benefit from a fingertip massage along the soft areas above and below his jawbone, from his ear lobes to the middle of his chin. This can include a gentle squeezing movement all the way along.

This will also massage the lymph glands situated in the neck, part of the lymphatic system whose function is to destroy bacteria and viruses.

See: Lymphatic system

jazz

The lilting, laid-back, syncopated rhythms of jazz lend themselves well to baby massage, provided the volume is kept to a moderate level. I have found that babies are especially partial to gentle boogie-woogie piano jazz, and the likes of Earl Hines, Erroll Garner and Jelly Roll Morton (who, incidentally, played in a trio with a man called Baby).

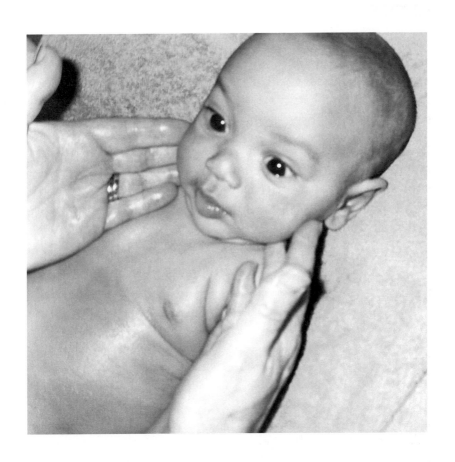

joints

Until your baby becomes mobile, he will only be able to exercise his joints by kicking his legs and waving his arms. As part of the massage routine you can encourage flexibility of his hips, knees and spine by moving him into positions similar to yoga poses.

It is good to continue this part of the routine with older babies and toddlers, especially as they may no longer be prepared to lie down for very long. Standing upright gradually compresses the spine and leg joints – this process can be counteracted by stretching and bending.

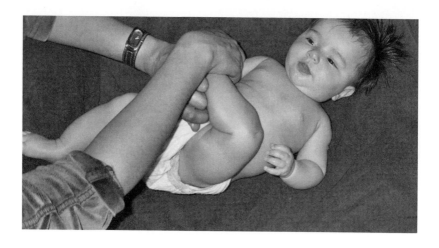

kicking

Kicking and arm waving are generally understood to be signs of recognition and enthusiasm in babies. It was accidentally discovered, in a labour ward, that all the babies responded this way when the theme tune to a popular soap came on the ward televisions; because the mothers had relaxed during pregnancy to this tv programme, it was also deduced that babies recognize the sounds they have heard while in the womb.

So don't be surprised if your baby is active and wriggles about while being massaged. It doesn't usually mean she is trying to get away, just a sign that she is eager to join in. You might want to rest your forearm against her knees while massaging her stomach, to keep them out of the way: being kicked vigorously in the stomach can be a hazard of baby massage!

kneading

This is an important massage technique, very similar to the kneading of dough for bread, when its purpose is to encourage elasticity by using just enough pressure to move the soft dough about in a push-pull motion.

Kneading can be done on any fleshy part of the body, and is especially useful on the stomach. Use first the heel of your hand (the lower part of the palm next to the wrist) and then the soft pads just below your fingertips, over and over. Position your hand sideways across your baby's tummy and make slow, firm movements, repeating them half a dozen times or so. This stroke is effective for constipation and wind.

kneeling

Some baby massage books and videos show babies being massaged by someone in a kneeling position with the baby lying on the floor. This may not be the best position in which to do baby massage, for these reasons:

You need to make sure that your back, most especially your lower spine, is supported so that your shoulders, arms and hands are relaxed.

If you are not completely comfortable you will pass on tension to your baby, who will not enjoy being massaged.

legs

Spend a bit longer massaging your baby's legs, especially when you first start. He will be able to watch what you are doing and figure out what massage is all about. If he wants to kick a lot, just massage one leg at a time. When you have finished massaging his legs, take hold of each ankle with your hands on top. Slowly cross each leg over into a cross-legged position and then hold the pose for a few moments.

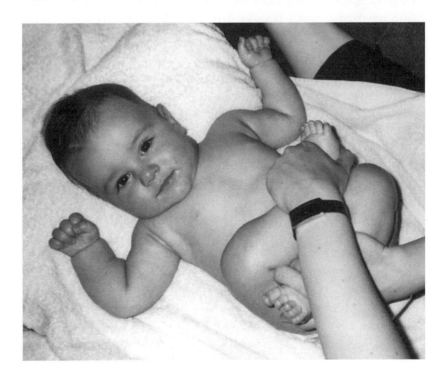

length of massage

How long should a massage last? The answer is that it all depends – on your baby. Some days you will be able to spend longer on his massage than other days. Twenty minutes is a good average length of time for a session, and longer is fine if your baby is enjoying it. There is no doubt that he will let you know when he has had enough.

In the classes babies may be massaged over a period of an hour or more, with breaks for feeding and taking a nap. Sometimes your baby will take a while to settle down into the slower pace of massage. He may need a time of 'unwinding' first, which can include having a cry. Because of the powerful effect of massage on the central nervous system, a shorter ten-minute massage is still beneficial, and well worth doing.

Really, though, baby massage is not a task to be completed but an encounter that takes its own shape and occupies its own space. You are entering a timeless zone, removed from the doings and workings of normal daily life. Forget about time for once – just see where it takes you.

lullaby

Like massage, singing is one of the age-old natural remedies for babies. Lullabies can become an effective part of your baby's bedtime routine, comforting and familiar, signalling the time to wind down, let go, and – with any luck – drop off to sleep.

It is characteristic of lullabies all over the world to be monotonous and repetitive rather than lively and uplifting. The mood of a lullaby tends towards the mournful – maybe they work because sleep is a pleasant escape!

New research at University College London claims that babies as young as two months old will "dance" to the rhythm of a lullaby; also that the lullaby is "training for conversation" and improves communication. If you like you can sing lullabies to your baby during his massage instead of playing music.

lymphatic system

Our bodies are mostly composed of water – or lymph fluid, to be precise. This fluid surrounds our cells and the spaces in between them. Its purpose is to destroy bacteria and viruses and to produce antibodies, so it forms an important part of our immune system.

Unlike blood, lymph fluid is not pumped around the body directly, but relies on movement to stimulate its flow. Before your baby can crawl and move around by himself, massage is beneficial for its influence on the lymphatic system.

Massage will also enable you to notice when your baby's lymph glands are swollen, indicating infection. These glands are situated in his neck below the ears, and in his armpits, elbows and groin; these areas require a gentle massage touch. Research shows that by 12 months of age massaged babies have better immunity to infection and need less medication.

massage for mother

Getting a massage while you are pregnant is an excellent way for you to relax and rest. Pregnancy massage is recommended up to and including labour. You can massage your own stomach with both hands, with or without oil. Stroke in a clockwise direction with a sweeping motion.

Massage can be done safely from the day after delivery – in India, mothers receive massage from the midwife for two weeks following the birth. Postnatal massage will help your spine and pelvis become realigned, tone muscles and promote recovery including healing from a caesarian delivery.

Massage therapists have told me that babies who are present during post-natal massage will generally relax alongside their mothers, and will often sleep throughout.

massage routine

It is not the aim of this book to teach baby massage in detail. There are some excellent books and videos that do this, and classes are useful for learning the amount of pressure to use.

In the meantime, using the illustrations shown in the next section, you can follow this basic routine to get your baby used to the different sensations of each technique.

Two minutes on each part will give you a 16 minute routine.

Feet: I like to begin with the feet, so the baby can watch.

Legs: Massage her legs separately, and then both together.

Stomach: Use your whole hand on her stomach, moving slowly.

Chest: Start at the shoulders to stroke down her chest and sides.

Arms: Slide along her arms, and then do each arm in turn.

Hands: Circle with your thumbs, and along each finger.

Head: Stroke her head and down the sides of her face.

Back: Massage her back as she lies on her stomach, or sits up.

massage techniques

There are a dozen or so techniques you can use on your baby, and of course you can invent your own strokes too. Some basic moves are outlined here; be sure to apply plenty of warm oil first, and only press on fleshy parts, never on bone.

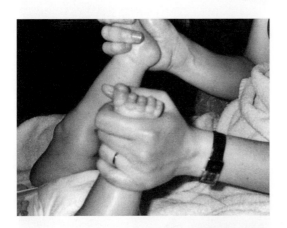

Enclose:

Wrap your hands around your baby's feet and hold them firmly so they begin to warm up.

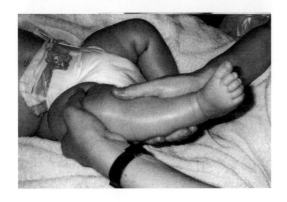

Squeeze:

Wrap both hands round her leg, one at the top the other below, and squeeze gently over and over.

Grab:

Grab hold of the fleshy part of the leg and squeeze.

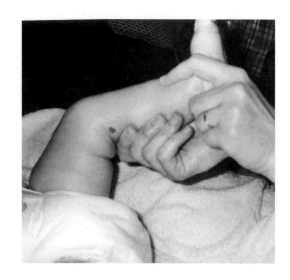

Slide:

Hold her leg at the ankle with one hand and slide your other hand up and down her leg.

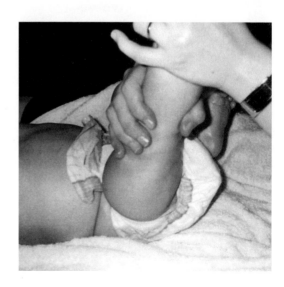

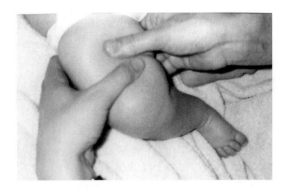

Stretch:

Move your thumbs apart to stretch the skin.

Stroke:

Long soft strokes down the length of the body.

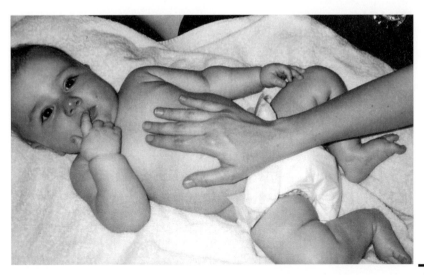

moon

Infancy, according to the astronomer Ptolemy, is governed by the moon. This theory was probably not derived from any direct experience of pacing the floor at night with a wakeful infant. Though, of course, it might.

multiple births

Baby massage is a great way to devote some individual attention to each baby, which can seem impossible with twins or triplets. Your babies may have to take it in turns to have their massage on different days, or you can get some help and run your own little massage session!   See: Twins

music

Classical music might seem the obvious choice to play during a massage session, but it has a tendency to vary in volume without warning, which can be startling. Meditation-type music is preferable, or recorded birdsong or ocean waves.

Different sounds have different effects: try an upbeat rhythm to start with, and a slower one to finish your session. I have found that babies respond with interest to the sound of flutes or panpipes, which tinkle with many higher pitch notes.

First Lesson

Lie back, daughter, let your head
be tipped back in the cup of my hand.
Gently, and I will hold you. Spread
your arms wide, lie out on the stream
and look high at the gulls. A dead-
man's-float is face down. You will dive
and swim soon enough where this tidewater
ebbs to the sea. Daugher, believe
me, when you tire on the long thrash
to your island, lie up, and survive.
As you float now, where I held you
and let go, remember when fear
cramps your heart what I told you:
lie gently and wide to the light-year
stars, lie back, and the sea will hold you.

> *Philip Booth*
> b. 1925

naked

Should your baby wear a nappy or not, for massage? This is an issue upon which the baby massage books and videos are largely silent, but it is a topic of interested debate in groups and classes! The decision is a personal one, so here are the pros and cons.

In the early days you may feel the hazards of your baby's unpredictable habits are such that you prefer to leave his nappy on to begin with, especially if you are outside your own home, and particularly if you have a boy since their range can be extensive! A good compromise is to loosen but not remove his nappy, so that you can replace it quickly if need be.

All the same, it is good to dispense with it when you can, so that you can massage freely and reach all parts of your baby's body. A nappy, for example, will conceal the lower half of his abdomen, so unless he is undressed you cannot properly massage this area with a circular stroke. A nappy will interrupt back massage, too, which should be one long smooth stroke from your baby's head right down to his heels.

I don't recommend massaging your baby directly on a waterproof surface. A large towel doubled over is enough to take care of unexpected wettings. In any case the towel will become oily, so it can go straight into the washing machine afterwards.

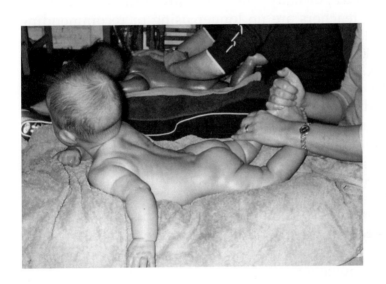

nut oils

In India babies are massaged with coconut oil. For some years I used this in my classes, but the upsurge of peanut allergy in children has given rise to alarm amongst parents about the use of *any* oil associated with nuts, although most of them are perfectly safe. As a precaution many baby massage teachers are no longer using or recommending coconut oil or even almond oil (the most common base oil for massage). Allergy organizations in the UK have given the following advice:

1. Neither peanuts nor coconuts are actually nuts: the peanut is a legume and the coconut is classified as a seed. Peanuts should not be given to a child under three years of age; this includes peanut butter and biscuits containing peanuts.

2. No link has been found with pregnancy diet in general, but if you have a family history of asthma, eczema or hayfever the advice is to avoid eating peanuts while pregnant.

3. If you need to check ingredients on food containers, peanut oil is also known as groundnut oil or arachis oil.

oils

The most suitable oils to use on your baby are fruit oils (grapeseed) vegetable oils (olive) or flower seed oils (sunflower). These are all pure, unscented, edible, and easily absorbed by your baby's skin without harm.

Some baby massage products contain a long list of ingredients, among them petro-chemicals and perfume, which may cause a reaction on delicate skin, or when ingested if your baby sucks her fingers. Aromatherapists do not recommend essential oils on a baby's skin before six months of age, although you can use them in a diffuser in the room while you massage.

Apply plenty of oil when massaging (except on the face when you should wipe your hands on a towel first to remove most of the oil). If you use insufficient oil there will be friction between your hands and your baby's skin, which is uncomfortable. Warm up the oil by rubbing it in your hands before applying it; in winter you can use a warmed bowl or container. And of course, warm your hands before you start.

The above oils are beneficial for dry skin and can be massaged into the scalp to relieve cradle cap. If your baby has eczema you can use the cream or ointment you have been prescribed by your doctor instead of oil (i.e. aqueous or emulsifying cream, but *not* cortisone or steroid cream which should be used very sparingly).

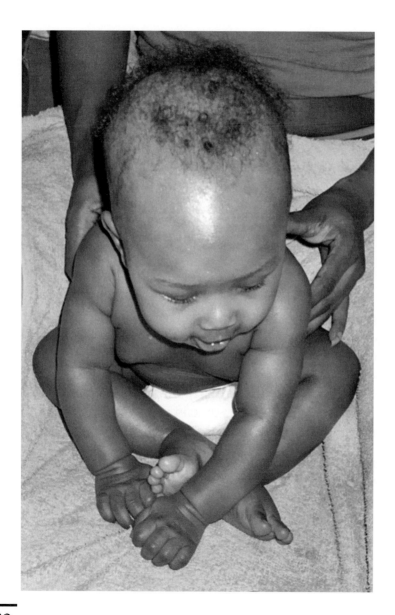

older babies & children

In theory there is no reason why massage should come to an end as long as you and your child enjoy it, but you will probably need to adapt the routine to suit a more active baby who may, for example, become resistant to lying down on her back.

Older babies can be massaged sitting up, and may be persuaded to sit still longer if they have toys to play with. Toddlers and older children may have watched you massage your baby and want to have a turn at being massaged too. It can be very effective just to massage a child's feet and hands.

In 1996 a Swedish massage therapist, Solveig Berggren, started teaching primary school children in Gothenburg how to massage each other's shoulders and heads; it had a calming effect on their behaviour, reducing aggression and improving their concentration. There is no reason why your children should not massage you in return: your hands, shoulders, face and head can all be made to relax by little fingers.

See: Baby story - older babies

older babies

Baby massage classes usually have a cut-off age, which is the time when a baby starts to crawl. This is purely because of the logistics of the classroom and the constraints of teaching a group, but there is no reason at all to stop massaging your baby just because he has started to move about independently.

Forward and backward bends (See: Pumpkin and Banana) and other flexing and stretching actions are fun for an older baby or toddler, and you can include some more passive stroking and squeezing massage moves in between them.

Jamil, aged four, would ask his mother to rub his back when he was feeling upset about something. Massage can help toddlers and young children to handle their difficult emotions; it does not have to involve the whole body, or oil, just some repetitive stroking through clothes. Head, neck and back can be very soothing, or try just feet or hands. Massaging the sinus areas on the face can relieve glue ear and congestion due to colds.

baby story

Judy's daughter Sasha started to have night terrors at the age of three, crying out in her sleep and waking her parents and baby sister. Judy discovered by experimenting that a simple massage of Sasha's feet while she was still asleep was enough to calm her. After doing this foot massage a few times the night terrors stopped completely.

At an orphanage in northern Thailand I worked with a group of one-year-olds who were only just starting to run about. One little boy was particularly demanding and aggressive towards the other children. Later when he was lying down on the play mat I sat beside him and started to stroke his bare feet. He became very still, but once or twice sat up to watch what I was doing, with an amazed expression on his face, and then lay down again, which I took as permission to continue. We had no language in common: I spoke little Thai and he spoke even less, but he responded well to the massage.

playtime

When your baby has been fed and changed, is wide-awake and wants nothing more than to play with you – this is the ideal time for baby massage. Although some soothing strokes at your baby's bedtime can be part of his 'winding down' routine, a proper massage then is not always a good idea, even if he seems to be wide awake and ready to play. For one thing you may be tired yourself at this point; for another, massage is stimulating and may enliven your baby rather than sending him to sleep.

Choose a time of day when you *both* want to play.

positions

When you have recently given birth, your back and hips are in a vulnerable condition, and need to be properly supported at all times to avoid strain and damage. If you don't already have backache, you soon will if you attempt to massage your baby in the wrong position.

The easiest and safest place to massage your baby is on the floor. Sit with your lower back right up against a wall or other solid support, so that the rest of your back, and also your shoulders, arms and hands are all relaxed. In this position you should be able to lean quite a long way forward without any strain.

Place your baby on a pillow covered with a towel, and put the pillow either on your outstretched legs, or on the floor between your legs, depending on which is more comfortable for you. With the first position you will need a small cushion or rolled up towel across your ankles to keep the pillow level, otherwise your baby's head will be sloping downwards, making it hard for him to see you. If your hips are quite flexible you might prefer to sit cross-legged.

If you find sitting on the floor uncomfortable, another position that works is to stand at a waist-height table with your baby on a pillow as above. If the table is too low you will strain your back by leaning forward. It is worth experimenting to find the most comfortable position.

post-natal depression

See: Depression

premature babies

Premature babies are kept in hospital until they have reached an acceptable body weight. When a group of premature babies was given a daily massage for ten days, they gained 47% more weight than a group of non-massaged babies, and were discharged from hospital almost a week earlier. As well as weight gain, these babies were more alert and active than the other group.

In many hospitals, nurses now massage premature babies, and encourage parents to participate.

pressure

The pressure used for baby massage is important – research has shown that babies who were massaged lightly did not gain weight or develop as fast as those who were correctly massaged. The appropriate pressure to use for a baby is one thing you can't learn from a book – including this one. I always demonstrate this at the start of a class, and people are usually surprised by the firmness of the pressure.

Too light a touch will irritate or tickle, to which the normal response is tensing up rather than relaxing. Babies respond well to the firm definite strokes of massage, which manipulate the muscles beneath the skin rather than just stroking the surface. A massage routine will include a mixture of firm and gentler strokes, finishing with a light stroke known as 'feathering', which tells your baby you have reached the end.

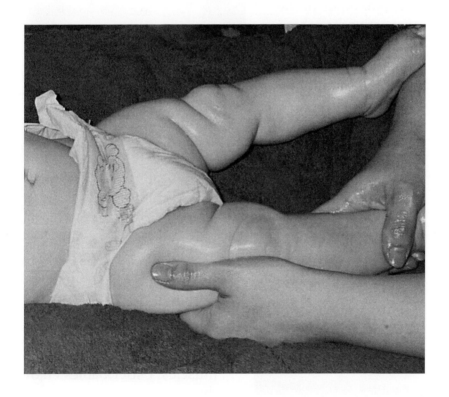

pumpkin

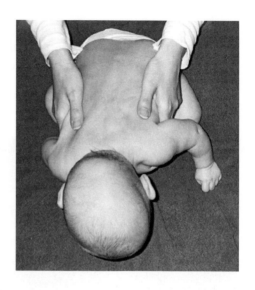

This is another of the more active stretching exercises you can do with your baby from three or four months, as part of his massage routine.

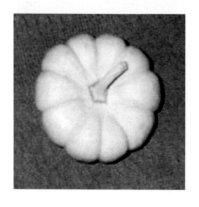

The plump rounded curl of your baby's back gives this exercise its name. The Pumpkin is a good partner to the Banana, which is a backwards bend stretching the chest, ribs and stomach muscles. Older babies enjoy these exercises.

Sit him up with his back to you, and place the soles of his feet together. The first time you introduce this exercise, gently coax him to lean forward as far as he wants to by holding one hand against his forehead and the other on his back. Keep your hands around him so that you can pull him up again after a few seconds.

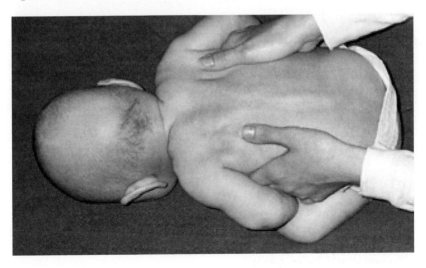

questions

These are some of the questions I am most often asked about baby massage:

Q.   When is the best time to give my baby a massage?

A.   Playtime, when your baby is wide-awake, not hungry and not sleepy.

Q.   How long should I massage my baby for each time?

A.   20 minutes is probably about average, but you can continue for longer if your baby seems happy. However, a short 10-minute session is not a waste of time, as this will still have a powerful effect on the nervous system.

Q.   What can I do if my baby won't lie down?

A.   Older babies may be unwilling to lie down for long when they are awake. You can massage her sitting up instead – lean her forward onto your hand to massage her back, for example.

Q.   How soon can I massage her after a feed?

A.   10 minutes or so should be long enough.

Q. What if my baby falls asleep during her massage?

A. This can happen even if you choose a time when your baby is wide-awake, but it will probably be only a short nap. Wrap her in the towel to sleep for a while, and continue the massage when she wakes.

Q. The first time I massaged my baby she cried – are there some babies who just don't like being massaged?

A. Not all babies immediately take to massage – if it is a new activity for you and your baby it can take time to get it going. Don't give up if your baby cries: comfort her with a cuddle and then try again. Your baby may relax better at first with a folded towel placed across her middle while you massage her legs and arms, until she gets used to the feeling of being uncovered.

See: Baby story - crying

quiet

Babies don't seem to enjoy a totally quiet atmosphere, probably because before birth they have been literally surrounded by a constant sound system. They are also able to hear noises that are outside the womb. 'White noise' such as a washing machine, or the car engine while travelling, is a very effective lullaby for most babies.

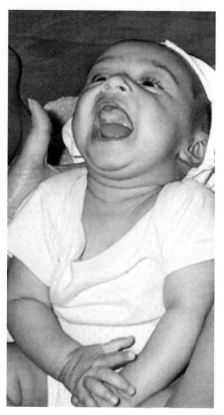

During a massage session, if you and your baby are alone, a certain amount of background sound will help to entertain and distract her.

See: Music

recovery from labour

According to Chinese medicine it takes two years for a woman's body to recover fully from labour. In Ghana they apply a rule of thumb to the spacing of their children: a child must be able to walk independently before another pregnancy begins, giving a natural two year gap between labours.

Researchers at the University of Wolverhampton found that a baby's adrenalin levels at birth can be a hundred times higher than those of an adult. Stress hormones such as adrenalin and cortisol are reduced by massage, while others such as serotonin (our natural painkiller) and oxytocin (the bonding hormone also produced by breastfeeding) are boosted.

Massage reduces anxiety in babies. The person massaging also experiences a lower heart rate and blood pressure. A similar effect has been found in elderly people who have a pet to care for and stroke, following surgery or bereavement.

resuscitation

It takes less than half a day to learn how to save your baby's life if he stops breathing, or starts to choke. Free courses are run at community centres and clinics, or you can request a teacher from the Royal Life Saving Society.

room temperature

At night your baby's room temperature should be between 16 and 20C (61 to 68F). Use a room thermometer, or otherwise check your baby is warm by touching his stomach. Because babies do not have good temperature regulation, overheating is a health hazard, increasing the risk of Sudden Infant Death Syndrome (cot death).

For massage the room should be warm and airy, but not hot. Remember that a big room with high ceilings can feel chilly even in warm weather. If the temperature is too low your baby will not enjoy his massage. There are two ways to check that the room is warm enough. One is by noticing how warm you feel in your clothes whilst remembering that your baby won't be wearing any: all but the lightest of clothing should feel uncomfortable.

The other is to check if your baby's hands and feet are warm or cold at the start of the massage, and again later. Babies often have cold feet and hands, even in summer, because their circulation is not very good. Massage increases the circulation and brings warm blood flow to the extremities, so if his feet and hands have not warmed up and remained warm after a few minutes, your room is probably too cool.

The exception to this is babies with eczema. See: Eczema

sensitive babies

Research psychologists have identified a trait they call "high sensitivity" in 15 to 20% of us. These people typically have a heightened awareness of their surroundings and are more affected and upset by certain conditions such as temperature, noise or light, which cause over-stimulation.

When this trait occurs in babies they are more difficult to care for in every way. They startle easily and can become upset for no obvious reason, may need to be held or carried in one particular way and be hard to soothe. These babies can have intense crying spells in response to quite small changes, such as being dressed or undressed, being laid down or placed into their car seat. They are likely to have irregular feeding and sleeping patterns, resulting in exhaustion for you and also for them, increasing the cycle of irritation.

If massage is difficult at first, try these adaptations: hold her in your arms while you massage just her feet, until she becomes used to this kind of touch. Build up the strokes gradually, concentrating on those she accepts without protest, and only for a few minutes at first.

Keep her clothed, or cover her with a warm towel or blanket during massage, as exposed skin can be unsettling for a sensitive baby. Talk soothingly to her and be ready to stop if she cries.

sensitive

It is often the case that you don't realize you have a sensitive or fussy baby until you have spent time with other people and their babies; first time parents may assume all babies are as difficult, and struggle on looking for solutions to the crying or lack of sleep.

When Fiona came to a class with Joshua he cried so much that she eventually took him out of the room so we could continue; later I found her in tears on the stairs. She told me about her feelings of disappointment at "missing out" on baby activities such as this class, anger sometimes at Joshua because she had no idea what he wanted or needed, and feelings of failure and exhaustion. From her description of his behaviour, it was clear he was a sensitive baby.

Joanne's daughter Sophie was her fourth child, but was quite different from her other three, and all her experience did not help her to understand Sophie's frequent screaming and her apparent misery. She would only accept massage on her feet and legs, and would cry loudly if Joanne tried to massage her stomach or arms. A cranial osteopath had been consulted for colic, but told Joanne he didn't think Sophie had colic, or any digestive trouble.

baby story

Having spent time with these and many more such hard to please babies, it seems to me that some babies simply do not enjoy being babies. Even when not crying they have a characteristically solemn, even glum, facial expression, all the more obvious when surrounded by babies who are quick to respond to a smile, and who often gurgle contentedly or even giggle while being massaged.

However, being persistent and patient with baby massage can pay off. The process will be slower and more gradual, as your baby may only accept being stroked on one particular place at first; the thing to do is repeat this as often as you can, along with lots of soothing and cuddling in between, and keep the rest of her body wrapped or covered.

It might be a matter of weeks before your baby is fully massaged, but this gentle 'desensitization' will help her learn to trust and relax, and become more comfortable with being touched. The effects of this process will be long lasting.

skin problems See: Eczema

sleep

Research has found that regularly massaged babies fall asleep in less than 10 minutes while the norm is around 22 minutes. If your baby falls asleep straight after her massage it might be tempting to think of massage as an instant remedy to use when she refuses to go to sleep, or when she wakes up in the night.

However, like exercise, massage releases brain chemicals called endorphins, which make us more alert. While regular massage can improve your baby's sleeping patterns over a period of time, it will not necessarily act as a reliable sleep potion and may, indeed, have the opposite effect sometimes.

Even if she does fall asleep afterwards this may be more in the nature of a short nap, after which she will be wide awake again. A massage in the morning will release tension by working on the central nervous system, thereby helping your baby relax and sleep later on when it is her bedtime.

sleep problems

For a baby the medical definition of "sleeping through the night" means a stretch of five hours. Babies in the same family can have very different sleeping patterns, and the pattern can change from month to month during the first year, as your baby grows.

Babies have a natural self-soothing instinct. Even when newborn your baby will turn and wriggle around until she gets her hand to her mouth to suck; this ability helps babies fall asleep on their own, and to settle again when they wake.

You can encourage good sleeping habits with a bedtime routine, and by reducing stimulation such as light, activity and physical contact. Even though very young babies fall asleep regardless of these, an older baby will not. If you think

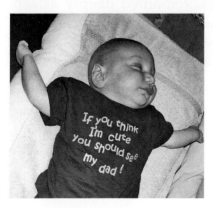

your baby is having sleep problems because she is in physical distress or discomfort a cranial osteopath may be able to resolve this problem.

sleep problems

We are mostly creatures of habit when it comes to sleeping – and habits are formed by repetition – so what your baby gets used to is what she will come to rely on.

Helen, for instance, encouraged her first baby to fall asleep by rocking him, and before long he would not sleep unless he was rocked. Having learnt from experience, Helen placed her daughter Katy in the cot to settle by herself, which she soon did. When you establish a bedtime routine, make sure it's one you won't mind repeating night after night.

All the same, babies can be baffling. At the weekly massage class Annie, aged ten weeks, remained deeply asleep. Her mother Maureen told us that Annie slept soundly throughout the day, and then woke up at night after everyone else had gone to bed, and became alert and playful.

Annie was Maureen 's third baby, and she was just as mystified as the rest of us. Neither of her other children had had this strange waking and sleeping pattern. Maureen said, "If I don't get up at night and play with her, at least a little bit, she just never sees me."

baby story

The only way to participate in the class was for Maureen to practise the massage strokes on her sleeping daughter, which she did, week after week. We were amused at the little curled up bundle whose repose was undisturbed by touch, laughter, music or the occasional crying of the other babies in the room.

At the fourth class Annie finally opened her eyes, stretched out and gave every appearance of being perfectly accustomed to baby massage. For the remaining classes she lay there quite content – and wide-awake – watching her mother or looking around the room. Maureen told us Annie had now fully switched to daytime waking and nighttime sleeping, and her family was able to get to know their new arrival properly at last.

slow down

One thing I frequently say in the baby massage class is *Slow down!* The tempo of massage is quite different from the pace of a busy day filled with tasks on a tick list, and this element of baby massage is just as important as using the right degree of pressure.

Life with a baby can so easily become a blur of activity and haste, and yet this time you have with your baby is all too brief; you will remember most fondly those times when you stopped to enjoy the moment far more than those days of getting things done.

There is a practical reason, too, for taking it slowly: your hands are big and your baby is small, so a massage of fifteen minutes or longer means lingering over the strokes, taking everything at a gentle pace, with much repetition.

Think of a fragrant soak in the bathtub compared to a quick shower; a stroll through bluebell woods to a trot round the supermarket; a leisurely summer picnic to fast food on the go. Like all these activities, baby massage can be rushed or savoured, timetabled or timeless.

stomach

The stomach should be massaged clockwise: this is the pathway of the large intestine. Massaging in this direction will therefore encourage the release of wind, and similarly helps with constipation, encouraging natural elimination.

A baby will sometimes cry when you first massage her stomach. It is a large area, within which a lot of activity takes place throughout the day. Your baby may feel unusually exposed at first – for a tiny baby it can help to cover her chest or legs with a towel to help her feel secure while you massage her stomach.

Other ways to calm your baby when you first start to massage her stomach are simply to rest your hand across the area without moving it at all, or to stroke the area through her clothing to begin with. Soothe her with your voice while you do this. It can take a while for babies to accept stomach massage. The stomach should always be massaged slowly.

See: Kneading

stress

When your baby is fractious and grizzling you might notice that she will quieten down when someone else takes her. This is not because she is angry with you, or because the other person is some kind of baby expert, but more to do with the fact that they are probably less stressed and frazzled than you are, so their heart rate and pulse are calmer.

The very close physical and emotional links between you and your baby mean she will pick up your mood and mirror your stress level. This explains why a baby so readily falls asleep on her father's chest as he dozes in front of the TV. One reason baby massage works better the more you practise it is because you too become calmer and more relaxed each time you do it. Your baby is sensitive to this, and so she responds likewise.

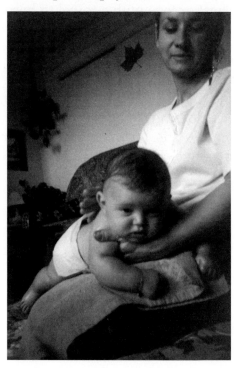

talking

From a very early age babies begin trying to talk, and will respond with interest to the sound of words long before understanding them. The tone of your voice will convey meaning all by itself; a baby who is spoken to will quickly come to recognize the different moods reflected by loudness, softness, humour, impatience and so on. Often, a baby used to the sound of voices will start to cry if he hears anger or shouting; even loud laughter can cause alarm.

If you maintain eye contact while smiling and talking in a soft voice, you may find your baby shows a surprising stillness and concentration, followed by a whole variety of little sounds as he attempts to copy the movements of your mouth. Talking one to one is soothing and intimate, like massage, and they go very well together.

teething

Because massage stimulates the hormone serotonin, which is our natural painkiller, it can help to reduce the pain of teething and provide some relief.

Try massaging your baby's gums by stroking firmly with your thumbs across his upper and lower jaw, above and below his mouth. The gums themselves can also be gently massaged with your finger.

time of day for massage

See: Playtime

tiredness

Massage has a stimulating effect on the central nervous system, and can be quite tiring for a baby. Some babies get cross when they are sleepy, crying loudly and struggling against it. If this should happen during the massage the only thing to do is wrap your baby in the towel and let him sleep. After a nap he may be willing to continue the massage.

You cannot massage your baby to sleep, nor is it good practice to massage a sleeping baby. Choose a time of day when he is not tired.

touch

Our need for touch is as great as our need for food, and babies who are fed but not touched fail to thrive. Research has shown that the less a baby is touched during his first three months, especially by his mother, the more anger the baby displays in mood and activities at the age of nine months.

But touch, although essential for your baby's growth and well-being, should be applied with consideration for his likes and dislikes. Your baby may not choose to have his face stroked, or he may refuse your attempts to stretch his arms out. He may enjoy his massage one day but resist it another day. This behaviour doesn't mean he doesn't like being touched, just that he has preferences.

The techniques of massage are not like medicines, to be administered for your baby's benefit, like it or not. Permission and a sensitive approach are needed. Your baby is entitled to his different moods, just like everyone else.

trauma

See: Birth trauma

twins

It's always fun to have twins in the baby massage class. Mothers of singletons are impressed and curious about how you manage two babies when even one is such a handful, and there is something fascinating about identical babies who can be very different in character and behaviour.

In one class we had two sets of twins. One set were particularly unusual, because they were so different; when they were born, three weeks before term, Molly weighed only 3 pounds while her brother Alfie was 7 pounds. There was still a very noticeable size difference at 14 weeks, as well as in temperament, Alfie being calm and placid while Molly was wriggly with a very loud yell whenever she wanted something. Being smaller, she required more frequent feeds and was more difficult to settle at night.

baby story

Both parents attended, taking each baby in turn, and over the course of the weekly classes Molly started to gain weight rapidly and to sleep much better. When one twin is more needy or demanding the other can be overlooked, so the class was a good opportunity for Alfie to get an equal share of individual attention from his parents.

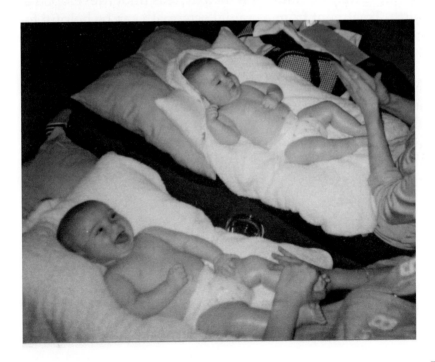

twins

Twins and triplets are often born before they are full term, either naturally or induced, and if they are very small they can have the same problems as other premature babies.

Their squashed position in the womb can leave them with tension in the neck, which aggravates the stomach nerves and may cause digestive problems or colic. Massage of the neck can help to release such tension.

Teething may be difficult if the palate is underdeveloped at birth. Treatment from a cranial osteopath can be helpful for this problem, and may also help when one or more babies have suffered trauma during delivery.

Multiple births put an extra strain on the mother's bones and muscles because of the additional weight and size, so that a longer time may be needed for full recovery. Parents of twins can find that baby massage is one of the best ways to ensure they spend time with each baby separately, even if the babies have to have their massages on different days.

umbilicus

If this area of your baby's stomach is swollen and protruding avoid massaging here until it is fully healed. You can still massage his stomach but work around the area.

ventouse

When I first started teaching baby massage in 1992 I saw quite a few babies with bruising around the temples caused by a forceps-assisted delivery. The pointy head that sometimes results from a ventouse, or suction cap, delivery has largely replaced this bruising.

This cone-shaped skull often sorts itself out without treatment. You can stroke your baby's head, including a gentle stroke across the fontanelle, without fear of doing damage.

I have also come across another problem caused by the powerful suction effect, which can have more serious consequences. The action of the ventouse can affect nerves associated with the baby's gut, which can result in feeding or swallowing difficulties that may be difficult to diagnose.

A cranial osteopath will be able to treat these problems safely.

See: Baby story - feeding

voice
See: Talking

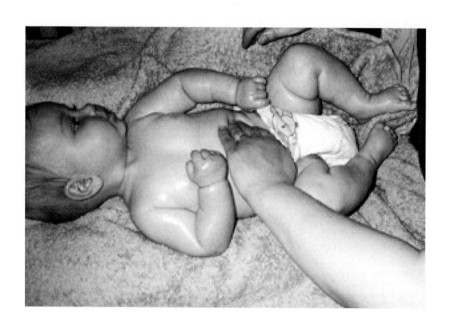

when to massage

For advice on when to massage your baby, see: Playtime
For advice on when not to massage, see: Contra-indications

wind

Massage is very helpful when your baby has wind, and there are a few moves in particular that usually do the trick. These are the ones we have found most effective in classes:

Knee bends   With your baby lying on her back, knees bent: take hold of her calves and press her knees into her stomach with three or four little pushes. This is not painful, but needs to be done firmly.

Pedalling   Lying on her back: 'pedal' each leg in turn

Waterwheel   Lying on her back: stroke down her stomach with one hand after the other in a paddling movement like the blades of a waterwheel. See also: Kneading

why massage your baby?

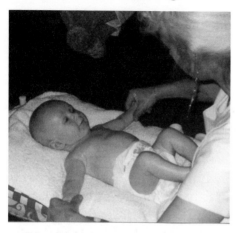

For a list of the beneficial effects of baby massage for both your baby and yourself, see: Health benefits.

A baby massage session can be a sociable event to share with friends and their babies; a family activity including your older children as well; or a special time to be alone with your baby – a little oasis of calm amidst the bustle of daily life.

Above all, though, it is for pleasure and fun – only massage your baby if you want to, and find it enjoyable.

xenoglossia

Xenoglossia is 'the ability to speak and understand a language one has never been taught'. Baby talk is xenoglossia: it has been found that mothers instinctively use a particular singsong tone with longer vowel sounds and exaggerated mouth movements, to which babies respond with rapt attention, and will attempt to copy.

Cryptophasia is another example: the private language that can develop between identical twins, which no-one else can comprehend.

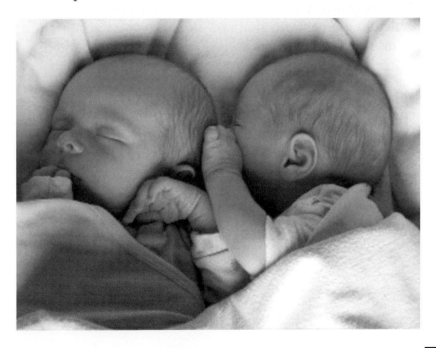

yawning

The natural yawning reflex relaxes the muscles in our jaw, and stimulates the tear ducts to lubricate our eyes. If your baby enjoys face massage encourage her to copy you by pretending to yawn, and then massage all around her jawbones.

yoga

Once you and your baby have got used to the basic baby massage routine, you can go beyond the passive techniques to include movements that are similar to yoga poses. These include forward and backward bends, arm wraps to 'give yourself a hug', and a version of the lotus position.

Your baby will achieve some of these positions all by herself when she is ready: pushing herself up on her hands with her head raised and back curved, for example, is a pose called the Cobra, helping the neck muscles to strengthen.

You will find these moves in baby massage books and videos, or you can simply invent your own, being guided by your baby's own inclinations. They are all versions of bending, stretching, rocking and crawling, and help the development of confidence and balance, as well as being a lot of fun. These moves can be continued after your baby starts crawling and walking, and they are a good way to harness some of the abundant energy with which toddlers are blessed!

See: Exercise
Banana
Pumpkin

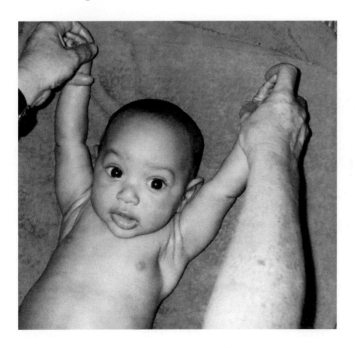

zugzwang

This is a term used in chess, referring to a blockade: a position in which any move is undesirable, yet some move must be made.

Zugzwang nicely describes the state you and your baby will be in by the end of an enjoyable session of baby massage – peaceful and contented, in a state of bliss – and at the same time thinking *what a pity we've got to get up now and do something else...*

That's zugzwang.

ZZZzzzz

Ideally, we would all get as much sleep as we want and need. Deliberate sleep deprivation is a recognized form of torture, and prolonged lack of sleep causes temporary insanity. Because babies are often the cause of our sleepless nights it is tempting to over-idealize the fast-asleep baby; however, sleep can occasionally be a symptom that needs attention.

Although rare, excessive sleeping or drowsiness in babies can indicate encephalitis or meningitis. More commonly, in cases of shock or trauma sleeping is a normal response of the nervous system, possibly as an escape or recovery mechanism. After a shock, for example, it is not unusual for a sleep reaction to set in, and longer periods of sleep often follow surgery or illness. In any case babies will tend to sleep a lot for the first two weeks to recover from birth.

In a limited way this response can be useful, but if you become aware that your baby is sleeping noticeably more than other babies by the age of six weeks, particularly during the daytime, it may be time to encourage him to be more wakeful, with some gentle stimulation.

Massage in itself has a stimulating effect; the technique for back massage in which you stroke *upwards* from the buttocks to the neck is enlivening and energizing; face and scalp massage are awakening, as are the more active movements described in Yoga.

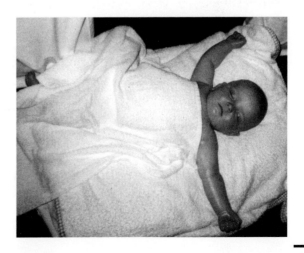

ZZZzzzz

Paul was born with a condition that involved a great deal of medical intervention immediately after he was born. The procedures continued for several weeks, and during this time Paul's parents went through great anxiety and stress.

Not surprisingly, at age three months Paul demanded a lot of comforting and physical contact when he was awake. The problem was that he rarely *was* awake, sleeping through the night but also for long periods of the day, a pattern his mother Karen only realized was unusual when she began to socialize with other mothers and their babies. She also noticed how often Paul cried during the little time he was awake.

It was difficult to wake Paul for his massage, and he seemed to resist waking even though he had been asleep for a long time when I arrived. It was almost as though, having spent a substantial part of his life in pain and discomfort, he now associated this with wakefulness, and was retreating into sleep.

I usually begin a teaching session with a short demonstration of the techniques and routine before handing the baby back to his mother or father to practise the strokes themselves. James held the now awake Paul who had started to cry

baby story

as soon as he opened his eyes. Eventually we settled Paul onto a pillow with his favourite music playing in the background, and I began to massage his feet, talking to him in a soothing voice the whole time.

Gradually Paul's crying changed to a less fearful but still uncertain wailing as I continued to massage his legs, chest and arms. After a while, Karen took my place, and she began to repeat the strokes on Paul's feet, talking to him as I had done, calmly and soothingly. Paul stopped crying and watched what was happening intently. And then something wonderful happened: quite unexpectedly he gave his mother a big smile - his first ever.

James and Karen decided there and then to give Paul a daily massage, seeing it as a way of offering him some pleasurable experiences to stay awake for. I showed them the stimulating back massage strokes that would help to energize and enliven him. From that first time with his mother, Paul continued to respond well to being massaged; meanwhile his sleeping and waking pattern gradually returned to normal.

I felt very privileged to have witnessed that smile.

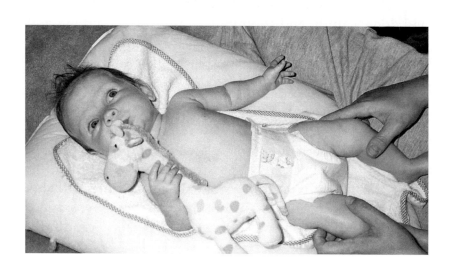

Afterword

Many's the time a mother has told me, as her baby joyfully responds to my smile or turns towards my voice, "Oh, he doesn't want to look at *me* any more!"

After working with babies of all ages for more than a decade, I have come to see that the process of separating begins much earlier than we expect; even at five months old your baby is a social being, eager to interact with his surroundings and with other people.

As natural and healthy as this is, seeing your baby's attention moving from you into the wider world is poignant, if not painful. Baby massage is a way to recapture some of the intensity you once had with your newborn.

When you and your baby become familiar with the massage routine, you will know that she is choosing to enjoy this special closeness with *you* just as much as you are choosing to initiate it.

Babyhood does not last very long.

Enjoy every moment!

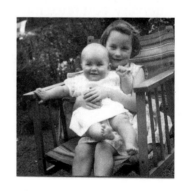

Booklist

There are many excellent baby massage books to choose from. Those listed here are the ones I found inspiring when I first began teaching, and which I consider to be the classics simply because they have been in print the longest.

Loving Hands by Frederick LeBoyer
Published by Editions du Seuil, France
and Knopf, USA in 1976
Newmarket Press, USA (paperback) 1997

Baby Massage by Amelia D. Auckett
Published by Hill of Content, Melbourne, Australia
1981 (reprinted 1989)

The Baby Massage Book by Tina Heinl
Published by Coventure Ltd, London
1982 (revised & reprinted 1993)

Infant Massage by Vimala Schneider McClure
Published by Bantam Doubleday Dell, USA
1982 (reprinted 2001)

Research sources

Comprehensive studies on the effects of infant massage which show:

- Premature babies gain weight faster
- Massaged babies fall asleep sooner
- Leads to improvement in eczema
- Reduces the stress response to inoculations
- Increases production of serotonin, effect on pain
- Improvement in asthma for older massaged children
- Health benefits for the person massaging the baby
- Amount of pressure for infant massage is important

Dr Tiffany Field, Professor of Paediatrics at the University of Miami Medical School, research carried out at the Touch Research Institute est. 1992

- The greater the mother's aversion to physical contact in the first 3 months, the more anger the baby displayed in mood and activities by 9 months

Dr Louise Bigger, quoted by Suzanne Adamson in Health Visitor Journal 1993

- Beneficial effects of infant massage after one year: strong immune system, less medication, better physical co-ordination than their age group, sociable and confident

  Suzanne Adamson, health visitor at Islington & Bloomsbury health authority, London, in Health Visitor Journal 1993

- Infants regularly massaged were ahead in neurological development by age 4 months

  Dr Ruth Rice, psychologist at the Newborn Behavioural Organisation, Dallas, USA, quoted in an article by Vimala McClure in the Massage & Bodywork Journal 1997

- Babies benefit from being exercised

  Dr Françoise Freedman, social anthropologist, University of Cambridge, based on her field study in the Amazon in 1978, reported in the Telegraph, London 1998

- In a controlled trial, baby massage helps mothers to recover from postnatal depression

  Dr Yvette Glover, Paediatrician at Queen Charlotte's hospital, quoted in the Times, London 1999

- Boy babies more physically and mentally vulnerable than girls; development 4-6 weeks behind girls; require extra care and attention in infancy; should be touched and cuddled more

Dr Sebastian Kraemer, Consultant Child & Adolescent Psychiatrist at the Tavistock Clinic & Whittington Hospital, London, in a report to Parent Child conference 2000

- At birth, babies' adrenalin levels can be 100 times higher than adult levels

  Researchers at The University of Wolverhampton's School of Health Sciences, 2001

- Babies show distress when eye contact withheld by mother

  Dr Robert Winston, Consultant Obstetrician at Hammersmith hospital, London: BBC television series on child development 2002

- Syndrome of the sensitive baby reported by:

  Meg Zweiback, Paediatric Nurse and Associate Clinical Professor of Nursing at University of California, San Francisco, USA: article published in Parents' Press 1998 titled "The Difficult Baby"

  and by:

  Elaine N. Aron in "The Highly Sensitive Child" published by Thorsons 2003